DIY HOMEMADE MEDICAL FACE MASK

Table of Contents

DIY HOMEMADE MEDICAL FACE MASK

INTRODUCTION

This database project base on the impact of COVID-19 in the world economy drawer medical mask with a single step, giving us more information about creating a cover, and the gap between the traveler and the people go on holiday.

The development of this book is to give people a better understanding of the impact of COVID-19 in the world and to overcome the challenges against this crisis, which have affected the world economy in general and have had a negative effect.

CHAPTER 1: 7 WAYS TO MAKE A CREATIVE FACE MASK

1. HOW TO MAKE A FACE MASK WITH A SOCK

Then we'll show you how to make a face mask with a sock in less than a minute, which we think is quite ideal if you are looking for an affordable alternative to buying a facial mask. All you need is a single sock (preferably clean) and a pair of scissors.

When it comes to making a facial mask, this method is undoubtedly one of the easiest (and one of our favorites). After all, most of us have a strange stalking sock at the bottom of our drawer mysteriously partner anywhere.

How to successfully perform a mask using a sock, follow these steps:

1. Take a clean sock and cut along the hose's width, a couple of inches below the heel.

2. Cut along the length of the sock, on the opposite side of the heel.

3. Bend your longitudinal hose, so that the top of his sock meets in which he made the first cut.

4. create a small incision on the fold line - this should be only a couple of centimeters long. You should find that you have created two small slits on both sides of the mask - these loop around the ears.

5. Try in the mask size, using the heel of the sock over the nose. For an additional layer of protection, we have seen many people place a folded part on paper towels inside his mask.

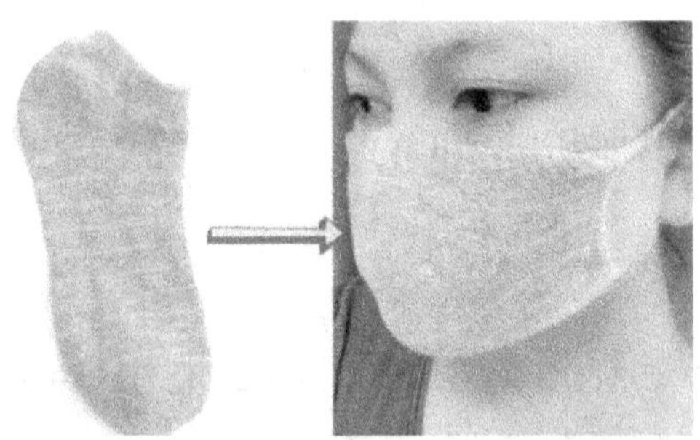

2. MAKING A FACE MASK WITH AN OLD T-SHIRT

Besides how easy it is to do, we also like the fact that you could just pop your shirt in the wash after a trip out to ensure adequate disinfection. This would reduce the risk of infection wearing masks.

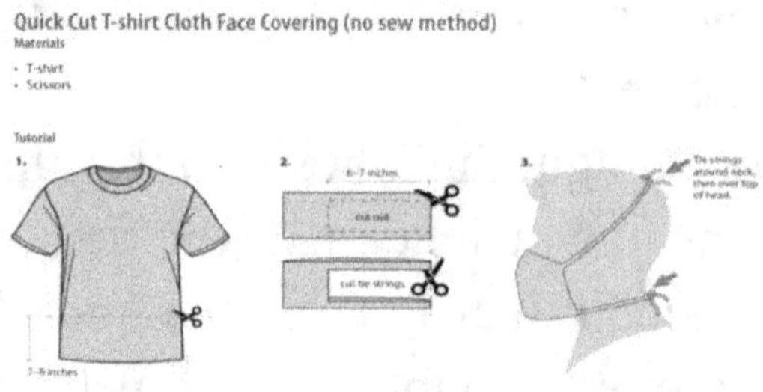

3. HOW TO MAKE A FACE MASK WITH A HANDKERCHIEF

This DIY mask without seams video tutorial could be the easiest we've seen. It is not only comfortable but fast, which means you can put your mask together in a minute or two if you are in a hurry.

All it requires is a handkerchief (a scarf or cloth large kitchen folded onto itself diagonally probably work well) and a pair of headbands.

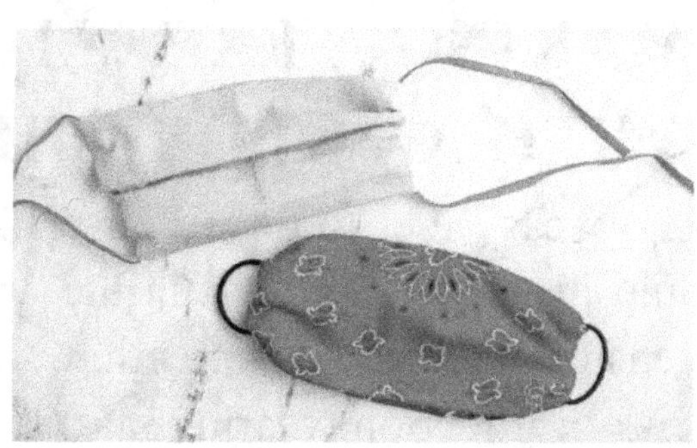

4. HOW TO MAKE A FACE MASK WITH A SCARF INFINITY

Infinity scarves are a better option worth considering if you are DIY-ing a face mask. It consists of lots of thin layers of fabric that can be wrapped tightly to your face without it becoming uncomfortable.

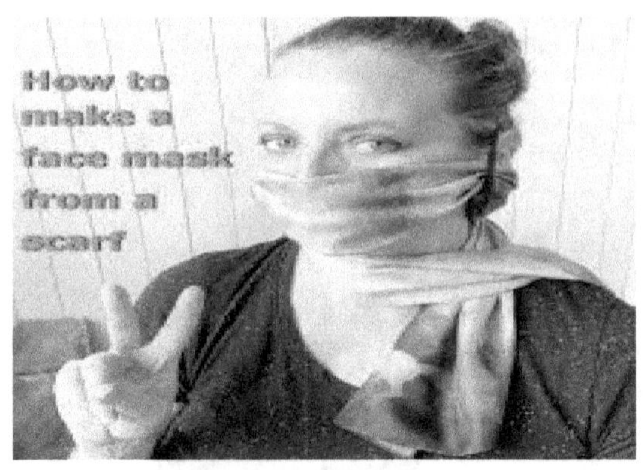

5. HOW TO MAKE A FACE MASK WITH A BUFF

While, unfortunately, none of us are going skiing in the short term, we might consider using an amateur like a face mask. We thought it might be one of the best choices if you are choosing to use a scarf as a makeshift mask.

They are very tight, which means you will not have to worry about crashing, but not restrict your breathing, because they are lightweight. Also, you can roll up to create multiple layers, which is similar to the approach we have seen applied to achieve many of the above options seamless.

You can also wash them in hot water wash, and will not lose its shape. They come in lots of colors and patterns, which can also be more attractive to children who are intimidated by the idea of wearing a face mask.

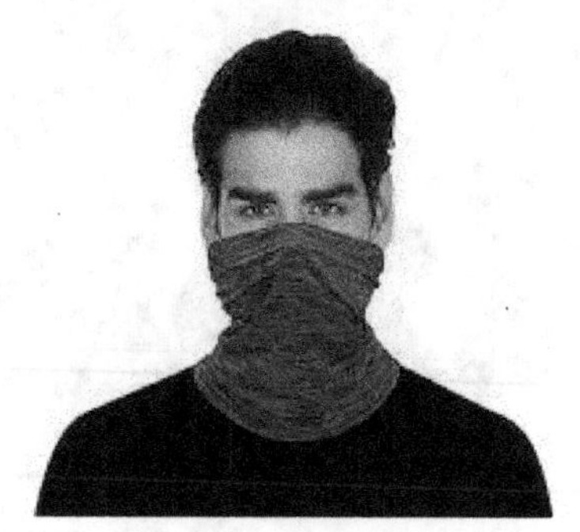

6. MAKING A MASK AND HEADBAND COMBO

Finally, this DIY mask without double seams like a headband, for example, I was walking to the store on the street with few people and only wanted to use his mask once inside.

The reason the mask is a social impulse

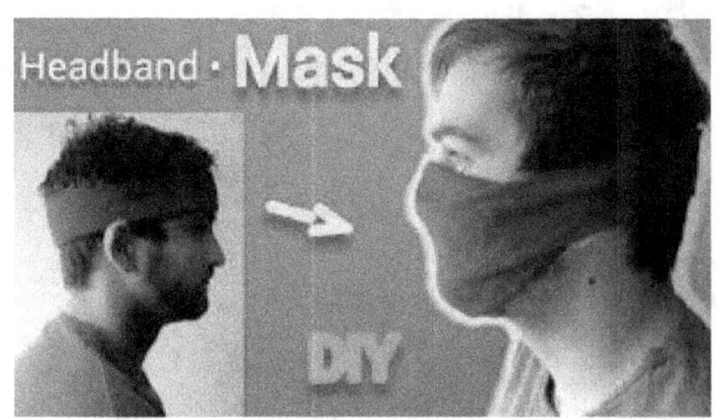

7. HOW TO MAKE A FACE MASK WITH SEWING MACHINE

1. **Cut the fabric.** For an adult size mask, cut one fabric rectangle 16″ long and 8.5″ wide. Cut two pieces of elastic, each 7″ long. Or, cut four fabric ties 18" long.
2. For a child-size mask, cut one fabric rectangle 14″ long and 6.5″ wide. Then, cut two elastic pieces, each 6 "long.
3. The upper side with an opening of the pocket. Fold the fabric in half, right side up.
4. Stitch along the 8.5 "wide edge, using a 5/8" seam. Leave a hole 3 "in the center of this seam to create so that the filter bag an opportunity, and to allow the mask is right side after sewing.

5. Press seam open. Zigzag along both sides of the suture by a cleaner edge.

6. Elastic tie pin or gender. Pin flexible piece on each side of the mask, an end at the upper corner, and one end to the bottom. When using tissue ties, pin a knot at each corner, with the rest of the lace sandwiched within the two layers of fabric.

7. Sew side. Sew the hands of the face mask—backstitch on the elastic ties or fabric for secure.

Cut corners, turn right on the mask, and press with an iron.

8. Sew Pleated Create three folds 1/2 "evenly spaced. Pin the folds in place, ensuring that all the creases are in the same direction. Sew each side to secure the folds.

Note: when the mask is worn, pleats are open downwardly to prevent the collection of particles in the folding pockets.

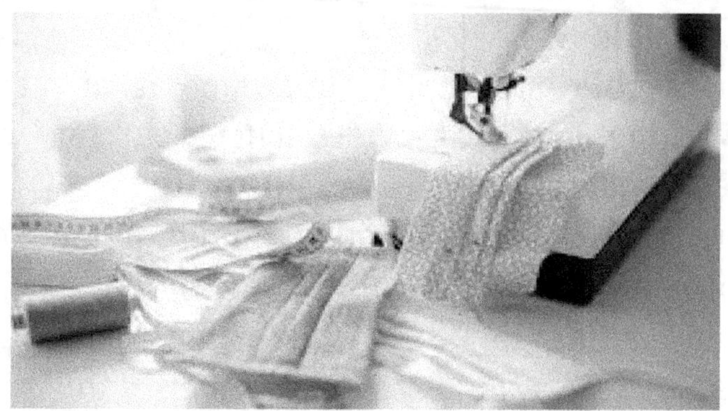

CHAPTER 2: THE REASON WHY THE FACE MASK IS A SOCIAL BOOST

WASHINGTON, DC - orientation of public health officials on how to avoid exposure to the new coronavirus has evolved over the crisis in the U.S.

Initially, counseling focused on handwashing, but more recently, authorities have urged Americans to wear face masks or covered in public. Consequently, an increasing number of Americans have adopted the use of masks to try to combat the spread of COVID-19. However, two recent studies by the Foundation Gallup / Knight show the new council seems to have introduced some confusion about the reasoning behind the recommendation to wear face coverings in public.

In late February, at the initial stage of the outbreak, U.S. Surgeon General Dr. Jerome Adams implored Americans stocking up on masks, saying they are not effective in preventing the general public from catching the disease and the need to be saved for health workers on the front lines.

Along with the US Centers for Disease Control and Prevention (CDC), Adams encourages the public to wash their hands often and thoroughly change. In

March, 88% of Americans said handwashing is more effective than surgical masks using, most of the rest (11%) saying that they were equally effective.

But on April 3, the CDC backtracked on its guidelines for face, following growing evidence that symptomatic and asymptomatic carriers R.P. can transmit the virus more quickly than previously thought. The new recommendation called for the use of masks or face cloth covers for Americans when and unable to follow the patterns of social distancing to prevent the spread to others, including unknowingly infected carriers in public.

The Gallup poll 14-20 / April Knight Foundation finds a sharp drop in the percentage of American adults who say hand washing is more efficient at 68%, and a concomitant increase in the rate that says handwashing and the use of masks are equally valid.

While changing patterns have introduced some confusion, the degree of change in all key demographic subgroups (including party identification, the communication media diet, and the amount of news consumption) is not substantial.

Notably, however, the opinions of older Americans are more likely to have changed. At the same time, younger adults remain hopeful that before I say handwashing is more effective in preventing wearing a mask.

Face mask habits of Americans

A separate survey question asked Americans how often they wore a mask covering the face or when they are in public in the last seven days. Those who have left their home in the previous seven days, on average to say he always wore a mask in general (36%), sometimes did (32%), and never did (31%).

In line with the findings of other surveys that ask about the face-covering Habits, Democrats, women, and people with higher education levels tend to say "always" or "sometimes" wore a mask over the last seven days.

Beyond these demographic differences, some other factors are correlated with the use of masks. For example, American adults who are users of heavy news, those who say they trust scientists and journalists "a lot", and those who live in a county that has recorded the deaths of at the least one of coronavirus related are more likely than their counterparts to say they always or sometimes wearing a mask in public in the last seven days.

In the same way, Americans who they think that wearing one is a mask as effective as hand washing in preventing healthy people from getting COVID-19 are more likely to say they had a face that covers the last seven days, compared to those who believe handwashing is more effective (75% vs. 66%).

Adhering to the CDC recommendation to wear masks is more evident among older Americans who believe that wearing a mask is as effective as hand washing.

bottom line

The American medical community's guidelines cover how Turnabout changed between March and April as new information emerged about the prevalence of symptomatic and asymptomatic P.R. and how the virus can spread.

The motivation behind the change in the orientation focused on preventing the spread of the virus by carriers. Still, the announcement has introduced some confusion about why people should wear masks.

Some members of the public seem to have falsely inferred that also implies that wearing a mask is an effective way to prevent healthy people from getting the disease. Yet there is no definitive scientific evidence to support or refute this.

Nevertheless, the announcement of these new guidelines was able to increase the use of masks in public spaces. Today, the majority of Americans say they always or sometimes wear a mask in public, especially those who consume a lot of new and trust the professionals such as scientists and journalists.

American social observation Remoteness less frequently.

Several states have begun to relax their social distancing guidelines regularly, while others have extended shelter requirements on site in May. Last week, 59% of Americans said that in the previous 24 hours, they "always" practicing social distancing. This is similar to 60% the last week but down from 65% reported that 6-12 April. Distancing percentage "very often" has not changed much, now at 29%, but the rate adhering less frequently increased by 7% to 12%.

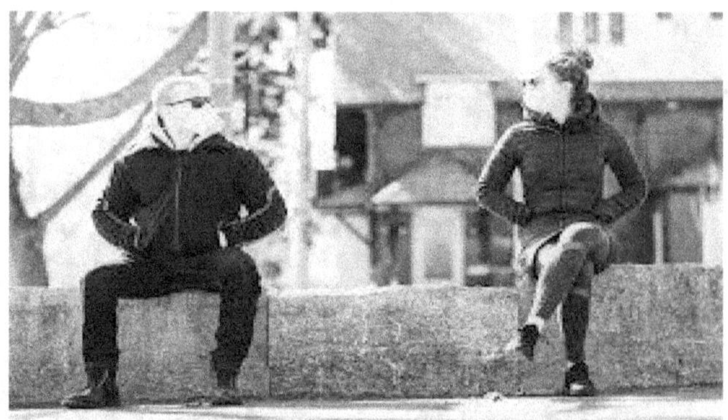

Most still avoid social situations in general.

At the least three-quarters of Americans, they say they have done each of the following components in the last seven days, while down slightly but still close to their April 30 March 5 senior Gallup interview.

86% avoided air travel and transit

80% avoided small gatherings of people, such as with friends and family

75% have avoided going to public places such as shops or restaurants

Also, 75% of Americans report now they have worn a mask on their face outside their home. This represents a 64% increase in the previous week and 51% in the first measuring Gallup, based on the 6-12 April interview. After joint discussion at the national level on whether the use of non-essential workers masks, April 3 the Centers for Disease Control officially recommended that almost all Americans wear cloth masks in public places where they cannot maintain social distancing guidelines.

CHAPTER 3: COVID-19 IMPACT ON THE WORLD ECONOMY

Since coronavirus spreads worldwide, states are grappling with finding the ideal strategy to address the global pandemic. In China, Singapore, South Korea, the U.S., the U.K., and Europe, different policies are a product of the State's capacity and the legal authority. Still, they also reveal competing views on the optimal role of centralized state authority, federalism, and the private sector.

While it is too early to know the long-term effects, the apparent ability of state authority centralized in China, South Korea, and Singapore to respond effectively and quickly made headlines in the U.S., the opposite was accurate.

The U.S. response is being shaped by its federal structure, a dynamic private sector, and culture of citizen participation. In the three weeks since the first U.S. case coronavirus, state leaders, public health institutions, companies, universities, and churches have been at the forefront of the efforts of the nation to mitigate its spread was confirmed.

Images security workers in hazmat suits disinfection offices of multinational corporations and university campuses populate the Facebook pages of America. The contrast with the efforts of the White House to manage the message, minimize, then quickly increase its estimate of the crisis is hard.

Puzzling response

For European viewers, the absence of a clear and focused response from the White House is puzzling. By the time Donald Trump President declared a national emergency, emergencies, and various State had was called, universities online learning had shifted, and churches began to close.

In contrast, in Italy, France, Spain, and Germany, the State directed national efforts to seal the borders and schools. In the U.K., schools are being opened primarily as prime minister. Boris Johnson has declared a defined strategy for herd immunity, which revolves around the exposure of populations resistant to the virus.

But the United States never shared the belief in Europe that the State should lead. The Centers for Disease Control and precaution., the leading national public health institute, and a federal U.S. agency have tried to establish a benchmark for the assessment of the crisis and advise the nation. But in this case, their response has been delayed due to flaws in the initial tests it came to deployment. The Federal Reserve has moved quickly for cutting interest rates and cut them back further this week.

But states were the true pioneers in the response of the United States. They had been using his authority to declare a state of emergency independent of the declaration of a national emergency. This has enabled countries to mobilize critical resources and the cities of pressure in action. After several days of delay and intense public pressure, the governor of New York, Andrew Cuomo, forced New York Mayor Bill de Blasio to close schools in the city.

State emergency declarations by individual states have given companies, universities, and churches the freedom and legitimacy to run and be ahead of the federal government to stop the spread in their communities.

Washington State was the first to declare a state of emergency. Amazon, one of the largest employers in the country, quickly announced a halt to all international and travel, and Microsoft, who donated $ 1 million to fund rapid emergency response based in Seattle. United have pushed their corporations to pioneer the response coronavirus sector. However, companies have voluntarily adopted the challenge, often getting ahead of state and federal action.

Google rushed to announce a move that allows employees to work from home after California declared a state of emergency. Facebook soon followed with an even stricter policy, insisting employees work from home. Both companies have also met with the World Health Organization (WHO) officials to discuss responses and predictable funding for the Solidarity Response Fund established WHO in collaboration with the Foundation U.N. and the Swiss Philanthropy Foundation.

Leading research universities in the U.S., with a unique position in the local public health and legal experience, have also been boosting prevention efforts. Explains just days after Washington, a state of emergency, the University of Washington was the first to announce the end of teaching in the classroom and online courses movement. A similar pattern followed in Stanford, Harvard, Princeton, and Columbia - each also following the declaration of a state of emergency.

Moreover, the Church of Latter-day Saints' decision to cancel their services worldwide continued declaration of a state of emergency Utah.

The hole in the U.S. response It has been the national government. President Trump's declaration of national emergency arrived late, and his decision to ban travel to Europe, but initially excluding the U.K., created uncertainty and concern that politics as much unity of the response of the House white as evidence.

This may change soon, as the House of Representatives has approved a bill COVID-19 response that the Senate will consider. These movements are vital to support public and private efforts to mobilize an effective response to a national and global crisis.

Need for public oversight

In the absence of better coordination and leadership of the center, the U.S. response it pales in comparison to China's dramatic moves to stop the spread. Chaos at airports in the United States shows the need for public oversight. As New York State Governor Cuomo declared the support of the federal government to build new hospitals, he said: 'I can not do it. It cannot be left to the states.

When it comes to global pandemics, we can discover that authoritarian states may have a short-term advantage. However, Iran's response and demonstrates that this is not the universal case. Eventually, registration of all authoritarian states as they tackle the coronavirus will become more evident and is likely to be mixed.

Open societies remain essential. Prevention requires innovation, creativity, the free exchange of information, and the ability to inspire and mobilize international cooperation. The State is undoubtedly necessary, but not sufficient by itself.

Efforts and resources of the State Department

The team of the State Department is working tirelessly to fight start

The State Department is taking decisive action to inform and protect U.S. citizens abroad, protect the homeland, promote the Administration's commitment to build global health security for this and future outbreaks, and reduce the impact on the U.S. companies and supply chains abroad.

We advise U.S. citizens to avoid all international travel due to the global impact of COVID-19.

Protecting the Homeland

The priority of the Department is to protect the United States and curb the spread of the virus. We have implemented travel restrictions prudent, together with our interagency partners, for people who have been present in areas considered high risk by health authorities in the United States. Traveling to protect U.S. citizens or live abroad, continually updated our travel warnings and alerts timely issuance of country-specific commuters to keep Americans informed and safe third.

Keeping U.S. Informed citizen travelers

The Department uses a wide range of instruments, including travel reviews and alerts to communicate the apparent security, fast, reliable, and safety information to help American citizens to make informed decisions about travel abroad. Every American embassy and the consulate has also updated its website to U.S. citizens in all countries of the world who have access to the latest details on Covid-19. We will continue to update this information frequently and encourage the United States.

Citizens read our latest opinions travel in their entirety and to register for receiving further updates Register Smart Traveler Program (STEP.state.gov).

Supporting the Labor Ministry and the preparation of our employees

The security and safety of our workforce are to departmental priorities. The ministry has issued interim guidelines on flexibilities leave and work for employees ordered or authorized departure and will update this advice is needed.

As a precautionary measure, the Department requested posts abroad to call their emergency action committees (CEC) to ensure the respective preparation after. The Office of Medical Services follows the recommendations of the CDC and WHO regarding the prevention, diagnosis, isolation, and treatment of all infectious diseases.

Support the response of the U.S. government

Assistant Secretary of State Stephen Begun directs the U.S. Department for his efforts on the White House coronavirus working group that coordinates and oversees the Administration's efforts to monitor, prevent, contain, and mitigate the spread of the virus. Experts from across the Department were mobilized by leveraging a wide range of stakeholders from the private sector bilateral, multilateral, and partners for a response consular, diplomatic, economic, and regional synchronized global Coordinating Unit Response coronavirus (CGRCU).

CHAPTER 4: OUR GLOBAL HEALTH LEADERSHIP

The White House appointed head of global health world-renowned physician and Ambassador Deborah Birx in the office of the Vice President with the whole of government response to Covid-19 as coordinator of coronaviruses interventions. Dr. Birx is exceptionally well equipped for this role, given his years of experience to lead the worldwide fight against HIV / AIDS as head of the President's Emergency Plan for the fight against AIDS Relief (PEPFAR).

Bring Home the Americans

Embassy Panama City staff work to help American citizens who return home on April 2, 2020. [State Department Photo / Public Domain]

The State Department increases to meet the critical challenge posed by the pandemic Covid-19, every day, everywhere.

The U.S. government has no excessive prime concern than protecting U.S. citizens. The State Department has launched a global effort to bring unprecedented citizens from all corners of the international and has repatriated thousands of Americans from several countries. Our organization is working around the clock in Washington and abroad, bring home thousands more in the coming days, from all regions of the world.

Helping U.S. citizens around the world

We perform to ensuring the safety of U.S. citizens abroad. In an exceptional effort, we repatriated tens of thousands of people in the United States in response to the epidemic Covid-19, in close coordination with the CDC and HHS public health experts. We continue to advocate U.S. citizens use commercial travel options and follow the advice of local authorities. We will continue working with our international partners to fight against the epidemic, help those who remain abroad and minimize risks for our citizens worldwide.

International Aid and Relations

President Trump's leadership, thanks to the generosity of the American people, has continued to demonstrate its international leadership in public health and humanitarian assistance in the face of the pandemic COVID-19. The management is deploying the full range of U.S. resources to contain and prevent the spread of COVID-19 at home and around the world.

Since the outbreak of COVID-19, the U.S. Government has committed more than $ 1 billion in foreign aid to date. This funding will improve public health education, health centers protect and increase laboratory, disease surveillance and rapid response capacity in more than 120 of the riskiest in the world of all countries to help contain the outbreaks before they reach our shores.

The State Department, USAID, and CDC are working together to support systems for health, humanitarian and economic assistance, security and stabilization efforts worldwide with $ 2.4 billion in charge of emergency funds Congress has appropriated.

The United States is by far the most generous and reliable partner to respond to the crisis and humanitarian action through UNICEF, the World Food Program, and many international organizations. Our leadership enables these organizations to combat the disease and, ultimately, protect Americans.

Americans not only assists with government media. We've helped populations affected by the pandemic COVID-19 around the world through the generosity of private companies, nonprofit groups, and faith-based organizations.

The United States has always stood by our partners through pandemics and crises. In the face of the COVID-19, the American people are here to help.

Collaboration with partners and allies

The Department is actively working with international partners and governments to combat the spread of the outbreak. Reaffirming the importance of diplomacy every step of the way, we have maintained close communication and close coordination with the countries concerned and implements the U.S. Government restrictions or problems advisory updates to ensure the necessary travel bilateral relations remain stable in the face of prudent and robust public health measures. The Government has informed the U.S. more than 100 officials from more than 70 nations.

We are also working with international public and private sector partners, including WHO, to rapidly improve our knowledge about the virus, our public health decisions, and accelerate research and development of vaccines, therapeutics, and diagnostics.

Building Global Health Security for the first line

The Department shares a global interest in the prevention, detection, and response to infectious disease threats at the source. The Department continues to promote the security agenda of the Global Health (GHSA) and coordinate the implementation of activities that help strengthen laboratories. Diagnostic equip front-line workers with the necessary tools and stocks to protect against outbreaks emerging, including this coronavirus

(COVID-19) outbreak. These associations have laid the groundwork to prepare quickly and effectively to emerging threats, including COVID-19. Investments in global security of U.S. health are one of the most effective ways to save lives and protect U.S. citizens from global pandemics and the spread of pathogens.

Mitigate the impacts International Business USA

The White House, the Department, and other government agencies are coordinating U.S. provide U.S. companies and employers with information about COVID-19. The Administration is monitoring the possible effects of COVID-19 supply chains and summon the pharmaceutical companies' leaders on the challenges of the supply chain that could affect the United States.

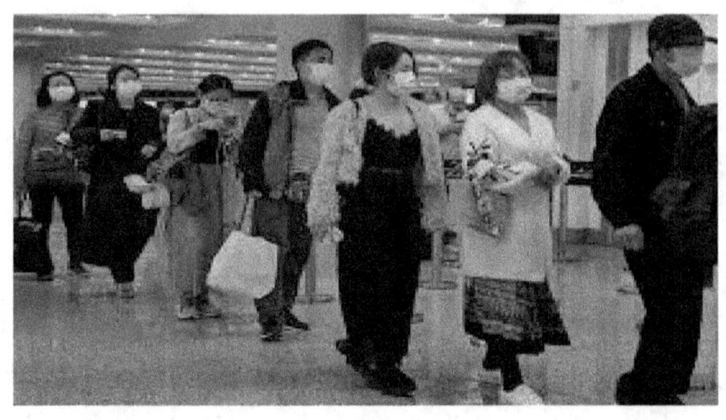

Promoting Transparency

The United States remains deeply concerned about information indicating that some government schemes may have suppressed vital details about the outbreak and, given the implications for public health, continues to reiterate that all countries transparently share information and cooperate with public health organizations and relevant international help.

The Centers for Disease Control and Prevention said Friday he had been mixing the test results of viral antibodies and on its website. The CDC says it is planning to separate those numbers in the coming weeks, but experts say that the current method is useless and potentially misleading.

This is because no antibody tests are used to diagnose a current infection or determine whether a person is potentially infectious. Instead, they indicate whether someone has been exposed to the virus in the past.

CDC spokeswoman Kristen Nordlund describes the practice of the agency told CNN on Thursday and confirmed the next day. "At the beginning, when CDC launched its much more common nationwide website and its reports laboratory test, viral tests (current infection) is used to serology tests (evidence of past infection)," he said an email.

"Now that serology tests more widely available, CDC is working to differentiate those tests for viral testing and report this information, differentiated by the type of test, published on our website COVID Data Tracker in the coming weeks."

Several pulses of antibodies and viral testing are combining up to the total number of experiments carried out in the USA. However, antibody tests are often intended for the general public - not just people with suspected infections - so it can skew a crucial indicator of how the pandemic is progressing: the percentage of positive tests.

CDC method also makes it appear that the U.S. has a higher capacity to test what it does, at least when it comes to identifying current infections.

"There is useful information unless you have a political agenda that you are trying to back up. That's the only reason to do that," he told CNN Medical Analyst Dr. Celine Gounder, professor of medicine and infectious diseases at the NYU School of Medicine.

CHAPTER 5: WHAT IS THE IMPACT OF CORONAVIRUS ON ECONOMY?

The impact of the coronavirus in the confidence of European companies remains limited.

Later this week will hit confidence figures for the Chinese economy for February.

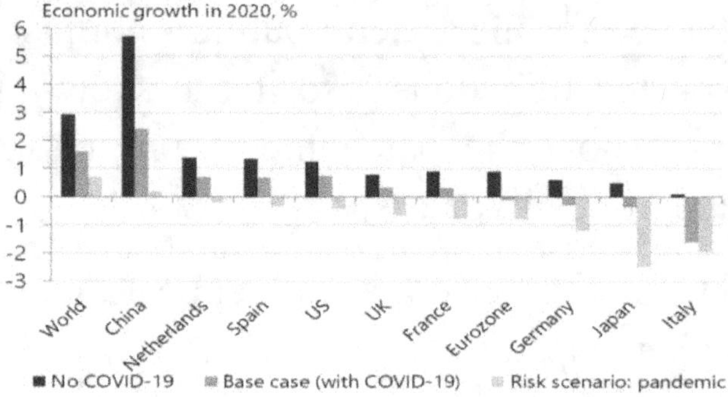

American consumers should continue to spend, and that's what we're planning.

Gold prices last week reached its highest level since March 2013. Traditionally, gold has performed well in times of uncertainty. The coronavirus causes the latter.

The rate at which the virus spreads appears to be declining slowly, but the epidemic is not yet content, much less. New cases in Italy testify to this.

We also have to see what will happen if the Chinese, at some point, to return en masse to work. Meanwhile, more and more companies undoubtedly supply problems and report production.

In any case, the first quarter of 2020 can be considered "lost" growth. China within a likely economic contraction compared to the last quarter of 2019, and worldwide growth halved.

The words of the President of Trump only add to the confusion She had told him last week that his reassurances were contradictory with prevention messages federal health authorities. This confusion in the letters of Washington has been pointed out by Democrats. Donald Trump accused of a hoax. When is the press that the questions themselves, denouncing the hysteria?

However, he continues. For example, recently gave a telephone interview with FOX News, the most-watched, three and a half million people s and their statements were then widely distributed.

Words truly amazing. First, he disputes the mortality rate of the WHO, and he said that these figures are wrong and that the virus kills far less than the claims of the World Health Organization. And to justify this charge, it is said to be his "hunch."

The President also believes that for many patients, the virus will be very smooth. And even he says better have to go to work. This is contradictory to the warning messages sent by the authorities, who recommend not going to work if you have symptoms. Donald Trump still obtained from Congress the release of more than $ 8 billion to deal with the crisis.

Coronavirus has little impact on the confidence of European business.

China PMI will scare the markets?

Next weekend, the office of Chinese official statistics (NBS) released its PMI (business confidence, measured by purchasing managers). These fully reflect the disorders associated with coronavirus. The fact is known, but it remains to be seen whether financial markets were spooked even more.

When investments go up?

In the U.S., we have paid particular attention to the willingness to invest in companies for a while. He played in a minor key. This was confirmed, for example, by small recent figures for loans in the industry. However, investments are essential if we want to achieve, as expected, about 2% economic growth for all of 2020.

On Thursday, we will receive the figures for durable goods orders for January. These figures are also an indication of the demand for capital goods. In recent months, new capital goods orders were below expectations. It will be a question of observing whether a turnaround is taking shape. Although, in this area too, coronavirus could (temporarily?) Confuse the issue.

We always count on the American consumer.

The U.S. consumer confidence seems to have been infected to date. This, of course, thanks to a stable job market and stock markets booming in recent weeks.

Dynamic spending nevertheless declined somewhat in the last quarter of 2019. Similarly, retail sales have been moderate in January. Perhaps because wage growth, despite labor shortages, remains limited. The average number of hours worked also seems to decrease somewhat.

Nevertheless, we still rely on the fact that Joe Six-Pack continues to support the U.S. economy. As investments - as stated above - do not restart, this support is particularly crucial. At the end of this week, personal income and spending for January will already give us an indication in this regard.

CHAPTER 6: THE IMPACT OF COVID-19 HAD ON TOURISM.

While the global financial crisis that began in 2007 in 2012 extends, its effects are felt everywhere: trust in banks slid, more families have no cash, and international migration is falling. Not unexpectedly, tourism has been affected as well, with a series of impacts at the national and international levels.

A 2010 report in The Journal of Research Travel, "The impacts of the global recession and economic crisis on tourism: North America," examines how the financial crisis affected Canada Travel, United States, and Mexico. The University of Colima, based on its report on multiple sets of data on tourism from 2004 to 2009.

In the USA:

In and in the United States, tourism has steadily declined in the year and a half after the 9/11 attacks. "In the six quarters advanced to the fourth quarter trough, the actual demand for travel fell by 9.5%. However, the real GDP of the nation increased by 1% during this period. "From that low point, the demand has grown at a rate of 3.7% per year to reach a new high in the third quarter of 2007. At the same time, the delayed real GDP growth at 2, 7% per year.

The current economic decline began in December 2007; in early 2009, the US GDP fell by nearly 4%, the worst drop since World War II.

In the first quarter of 2009, the actual demand for travel fell 6% over six quarters. "This decrease was far more gentle than what took place after the 9/11 attacks. But the decline was twice as fast as real GDP dropped.

"Tourism employment culminates at nearly 6 million jobs in the first quarter of 2008. Therefore, in the first quarter of 2009, more than 250,000 jobs were lost in the sector.

Even though the slight inflation continues, "travel prices have fallen twice as fast in the current recession as after the 9/11 attacks. "

In Mexico.

Despite natural disasters and ongoing issues with internal security from 2005 until the first half of 2008, international arrivals to Mexico rose to nearly 6% per year. However, there was a remarkable variation along the way, including drops of 5.35% in 2006 and 3.9% in 2007.

"The data [confirm] that there are other factors that have a major impact on the tourism industry in Mexico that the collapse of financial markets and economic activity."

The exchange rate between the peso and other currencies has a significant influence on the influx of foreign visitors. "Ironically, when the Mexican economy falters, and the peso depreciates, the benefits of the tourism sector and tourism services in Mexico are more affordable in the eyes of foreign visitors."

For Canada:

From 2007 to 2008, Canadian spending in the United States decreased by 15%, and spending the U.S. in Canada, declined by 6%.

In May 2009, international travelers made 1.4 million overnight trips to Canada, down 7% from the previous year.

Donald Trump said the United States would suspend all trips from Europe for 30 days from Friday.

Will Canada have to do the same with the United States?

The U.S. president said in a speech to the nation delivered Tuesday night.

The closure of the U.S. border, which will have significant consequences for the world economy, will be in effect from midnight on Friday. The United Kingdom is not affected by the measure.

Donald Trump has been attributed partly to blame Europe for the situation in his country, not to close their borders quickly to travelers from China or other countries affected by the virus.

At the moment, Canada is safe from this measure imposed by Trump. However, nothing is guaranteed, according to our columnist Bernard Ville drain.

A heavyweight

Most calculator's carbon footprint estimates that the use of a car adds about 2.5 tons of greenhouse gases for the balance of a person per 10,000 kilometers traveled. Leave your car at home to take public transportation can reduce the carbon footprint of a person by 26% to 76%, according to some studies.

"It is clear that the abandonment of the car is what has the most significant impact because it eliminates emissions due to the use of the vehicle, but also those linked to manufacturing, which is very important in terms of weight of carbon. 'A vehicle. This is why carpooling would be an effective solution, limiting the two sources of emissions associated with cars, more than carsharing, "adds MS Potvin.

Ineffective Gestures

Governments are multiplying campaigns and guides to encourage citizens to reduce their carbon footprint. However, according to a study conducted in 2017 at the University of Vancouver and the University of Lund in Sweden, most of the proposed actions by public officials are successful for relatively ineffective measures oriented to reduce greenhouse gases. Tight.

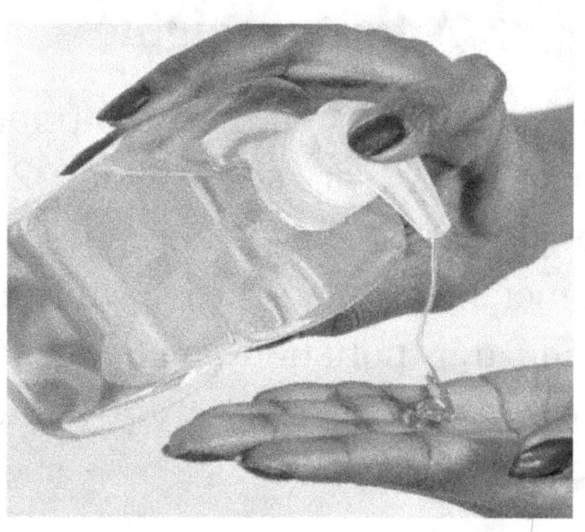

More than 148 proposed actions, the three countries with the carbon footprint highest per capita in the world (Canada, United Kingdom, and the United States), none suggests reducing air transport (between 0.7 and 3.2 tones of CO_2 per flight) or the benefits of a meatless diet (a discount of up to 1.6 tons per year).

Furthermore, various measures guides include a low impact on greenhouse gases, such as drying clothes to the outside (-0.21 tCO_2 / yr) or the laundry in cold water (-0.25 tCO_2 / year) more efficient measures to reduce your electricity bill gases associated with global warming.

Beneficial and direct solutions are often absent from public discourse, Catherine Potvin believes. Instead of adopting a guilty tone for the use of motorized transport, she said, she must promote solutions to avoid avoidable trips such as teleworking or Skype meetings.

"I think we need to look at other ways of doing things. We have the highest rate of emissions per person in the world, which seems to be reason enough to say that we have a long way to go. Indeed, in the regions, people often have no choice other than the car. And this is where governments must intervene. For the rest, it's like a diet, and we start by cutting where it hurts the least. "

It rings a new virus in China and rose to six dead, and more than 300 cases on Tuesday as millions of Chinese people are willing to travel for the Lunar New Year, which increases the risk of contagion.

Many in China are scrambling to buy masks to protect against coronavirus infection, such as influenza previously unknown and airports World tight screening.

The epidemic, which began in the central Chinese city of Wuhan, also concerned about the financial markets, investors recalled the economic consequences of a severe outbreak of severe acute respiratory syndrome (SARS) in China in 2002/2003 it initially covered.

The SARS coronavirus has killed nearly 800 people then.

"We will stay at home during the holidays. I'm afraid I vividly remember SARS, "said Zhang Xinyuan, which had been bound from Beijing to the Thai resort of Phuket before she and her husband definite to cancel their tickets.

Authorities confirmed more than 300 cases of new coronavirus in China, mostly in Wuhan, provincial capital and transportation hub, where it may come from a seafood market.

Manifestation includes fever, coughing and breathing difficulties, and viral infection can cause pneumonia.

Wuhan Mayor Zhou Xian Wang said Chinese state television Tuesday six people had died in his city. The disease is spreading around other parts of China, including five cases in the national capital Beijing.

"Fifteen medical personnel are among those illnesses."

Abroad, Thailand has reported two cases and South Korea, all involving Chinese Wuhan. Japan and Taiwan have confirmed one each incident, the two nationals who had been in Wuhan.

The World Health Organization (WHO) held a meeting on Wednesday to consider whether the epidemic is an international public health emergency.

Doctors and alarmed markets

"Information on new infections reported suggest it may be now sustained human transmission," said WHO Regional Director for the Western Pacific, Takeshi Kasai.

Taiwan, the island governed by saying that China claims as its own, set up an epidemic response center. Over 1,000 beds have been prepared in isolation wards in case the virus spreads further.

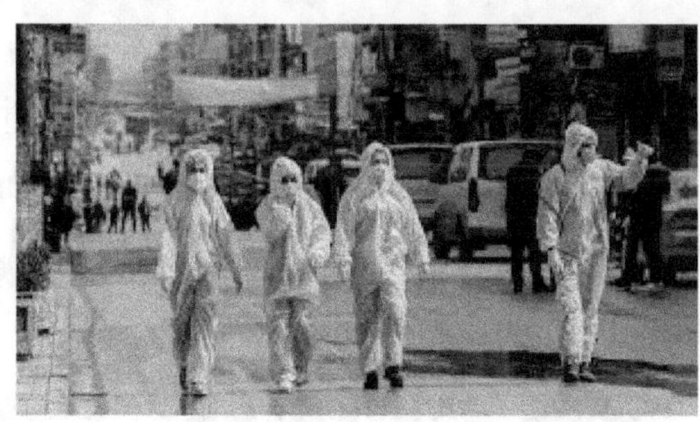

North Korea was to ban foreign tourists, who are mainly Chinese temporarily, an international tour operator said.

Fear agitated risk aversion in global markets, with Asia particularly affected.

Hong Kong, which has suffered much during the SARS outbreak, saw its index down 2.8%. Japan's Nikkei lost 0.9% and 1.7% blue-chip Shanghai, with the pressure airlines.

Coronavirus cases will increase as more people travel ahead of the Lunar New Year

In Europe, shares of luxury goods manufacturers, which have broad exposure to China, were among the most decline.

The Chinese yuan fell nearly 0.7% in offshore operations to 6.9126 per dollar, on land, which fell to its lowest level in more than a week at 6.9094.

Although the virus's origin has not yet been identified, WHO said it was probably the primary source of animal. Chinese officials have linked the outbreak of the Wuhan seafood market.

More functions and masks

"The outbreak of SARS coronavirus in Wuhan is becoming an important potential economic risk of the Asia-Pacific now that there is medical evidence of human to human transmission," said Rajiv Biswas, chief Asia Pacific economist at IHS mark it.

So far, WHO has not recommended travel restrictions or trade, but can be discussed on Wednesday. National Health Commission of China is also scheduled to give an update at a press conference at 10 a.m. on Wednesday.

Airports in the United States, Australia, and Asia have begun screening passengers extra Wuhan.

In the city itself, officials have been using ruddy thermometers to screen travelers at airports, railway stations, and other traveler terminals from January 14.

The Lunar New Year is an important holiday for the Chinese, many of whom travel to join the family or have a holiday abroad.

Long lines formed to buy masks in cities. Some online vendors selling masks and hand sanitizers limited because of the increased demand.

According to the publication on the website of Shanghai Observer, market regulator Shanghai city warned that punish speculators hoard masks or other products used for the prevention of infectious diseases.

Chinese travel booking platforms from to Fliggy Alibaba Group said they would offer free cancellations in bookings made for Wuhan, while South Korea's low-cost airline Air T'way postponed the launch of a new route to the city.

Zhong Nanshan, head of the team of the National Health Commission investigating the outbreak, aimed to improve alarm, saying in images shown on state television that there was no danger that the SARS epidemic repeat, as long as they take the precautions.

T'Way launch air is stopped due to virus concerns.

Due to the growing concern about the spread of a new coronavirus, South Korea's low-cost airline Air T'way has postponed the scheduled launch Tuesday of a new route to the Chinese city of Wuhan.

Monday, South Korea reported the first confirmed case of the illness from 35-year-old Chinese national who flew from Wuhan to Seoul on Sunday.

T'way was set for the first of two times a week from the central axis of Korea South Incheon to Wuhan at 1020 pm (1320 GMT), but canceled plans because of the epidemic, and the official said the company.

"It was an unavoidable decision because of the situation there," the official told Reuters, adding that it will closely monitor developments.

The decision came amid spiraling fears about the virus, which could spread through human contact with millions of Asians traveling on vacation the Lunar New Year this week. In China, the number of confirmed cases rose to 291 on Monday.

An official of the Korean Air Lines, the only other airline Korean Southern direct flights to Wuhan works, said the company has no plans to suspend its route four times running per week, but not to raise cancellation fees Tickets for travel to the city,

Centers South Korea for Disease Control and Prevention warned on Tuesday tourists from contact with animals and people showing respiratory symptoms and visits market in China.

President Moon Jae-in instructed local authorities to step up prevention efforts, with many South Koreans living in China. He expected to return home and some 32 million traveling around the country for vacation until next week.

FASHION NOW

Too little or too much money? Here's what the IRS said about inaccurate stimulus payments

Mitch McConnell Senate majority leader, R-KY,

The following Bill coronavirus is a "final," said Mitch McConnell

Here's how the unpaid debt is processed when a person dies

Protesters burn a flag outside the CNN Center on May 29, 2020, in Atlanta, Georgia. Events are held across the U.S. after George Floyd died in custody on May 25 in Minneapolis, Minnesota.

Protests and riots in cities in the U.S. that the bubbling anger after the assassination of George Floyd

A prototype rocket SpaceX Starship after a test explosion on May 29, 2020.

SpaceX prototype explodes the Starship rocket after the test in Texas

by commercial taboola.

The results of a new virus in China rose to six dead, and more than 300 cases on Tuesday as millions of Chinese people were willing to travel for the Lunar New Year, which increased the risk of contagion.

Many in China are scrambling to buy masks to protect against coronavirus infection, such as influenza previously unknown and airports World tight screening.

The epidemic, which began in the central Chinese city of Wuhan, also concerned about the financial markets, investors recalled the economic consequences of a severe outbreak of severe acute respiratory syndrome (SARS) in China in 2002/2003 it initially covered.

Symptoms include fever, coughing and breathing difficulties, and viral infection can cause pneumonia.

Wuhan Mayor Zhou Xian-wang said Chinese State television Tuesday six people had died in his city. The disease is spreading around other parts of China, including five cases in the international capital Beijing.

Fifteen medical personnel are among those infected.

Abroad, Thailand has reported two cases and South Korea, all involving Chinese Wuhan. Japan and Taiwan have confirmed one each incident, the two nationals who had been in Wuhan.

The World Health Organization (WHO) held a meeting on Wednesday to consider whether the epidemic is an international public health emergency.

"It was an inevitable decision because of the situation there," the official told Reuters, adding that he would continue to monitor developments.

The move came amid fears the virus rises sharply, which could be spread by human contact with millions of Asians traveling for the holidays Lunar New Year this week. In China, the number of confirmed cases rose to 291 Monday.

CHAPTER 7: HOW TO THINK OF TRAVEL AS IT EVOLVES THE CORONAVIRUS THREAT

(Enisaurus for the Washington Post)

By Hannah Sampson March 2,

Travelers could quickly adapt in the early days of the outbreak of coronavirus when the disease was contained mainly a province in China. Then they began to appear cases and spread in other countries.

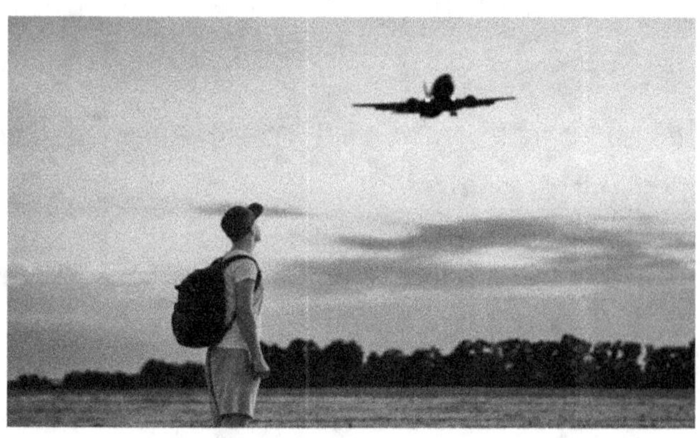

Concerns about the widespread disease in places like Italy anxieties brought closer to American travelers. Friday night, the U.S. State Department raised its warning level to warn Americans to reconsider travel throughout Italy due to "sustained community spread" of the virus. He warned not to travel in the regions of Lombardy and Veneto. More than 1,600 people have tested positive there. The Centers for Disease Control and Disease Prevention also raised its tongue over the country, issuing a warning to avoid all non-essential travel.

"I would not be predicted a week ago that northern Italy would be a place that can not travel at the moment would," Robert Quigley, regional medical director for risk mitigation travel company International SOS, said Thursday before warnings were lifted. "You can not predict where will be the next success."

Last week, authorities confirmed cases in the United States without known origin, which marks a new chapter for the spread in the country.

As each day brings news of more cases, which is a potential traveler to do?

Is it time to cancel a trip? Should people get on with their holiday and programadas-? And for those who still determined to travel, what is the best way to plan?

If you decide to cancel

Stay on the site is not a common practice in the past few days. Large corporations suspended large gatherings, and hotel chains reported increasing cancellations. Some travel agents say customers are canceling plans cruises abroad and changing US-based outputs or all-inclusive resorts. Like American Airlines, JetBlue and Alaska, waived cancellation and change fees for new customer bookings case get nervous about traveling.

Experts say there are potential resources. Travelers should consider deciding whether to call off a trip, including counseling and situation reports from the World Health Organization, warnings of the State Department, which often contain detailed information about specific regions within a country and communications CDC. From Monday the Food and Drug Administration warned the non-essential American travel to China, Iran, South Korea, and Italy, and improve the protection measures in Japan due to the corona to be avoided.

Few people are March 2 in Piazza Navona in Rome, which is usually full of tourists. Italy's tourism industry has been affected by the coronavirus outbreak, with hotel-reporting cancellations in droves, even in cities with few or no cases of the virus. (Remo Casilli / Reuters)

"I think right now, we see that more transmission in certain parts of the world, and so it is important to keep in mind where it was reported to transfer," said Crystal Watson, an assistant professor at Johns Hopkins University Center for Health, safety."Those places might not be the best places to go if you can avoid traveling there. But I that soon we will see a lot more transmission worldwide."

CHAPTER 8: THESE AIRLINES OFFER FLEXIBLE TRAVEL OPTIONS, ADAPT TO THE SPREAD OF THE CORONA.

To choose those who know what to do, said Watson should consider whether they are at a higher risk of serious illness if infected. This includes people over 65 and those with underlying health conditions.

Isaac Bogoch, an infectious disease physician and scientist at the University of Toronto, said that although the patterns so far show most people infected with coronavirus have mild symptoms, there are still many questions.

"I think we have to stay still modest as we do not have the answers," he said. "Because of this and because we do not have a vaccine and because we do not know a lot about this virus, people can have some fear wherever there are unknowns. "

Square mouth, the travel insurance comparison site, noted a "huge spike" in customer calls last week after the virus spread in Italy. According to a company survey offers, after people buy insurance, 27 percent said they purchased because of the coronavirus.

"Right now, we hear mainly customers who want to cancel their trip because they are worried about how the virus will spread, while the general feeling of fear and uncertainty," said the spokesman mouth square Kasara Barto. "Or they are still planning to travel, but they want to be able to buy a policy that allows them to cancel in case the epidemic spreads. "

Companies canceling U.S. domestic travel on fears coronavirus

Most booked and want to cancel because they are afraid to travel or because their primary reason for traveling may not be valid. They would be out of luck unless they purchased a comprehensive policy that allows them to call their travel for any reason.

Barto recommends calling hotels, airlines, and cruise lines to see if they can waive rebooking fees, change travel dates, or offer flexibility. Those who have booked a trip with a travel agent must consider whether this person can have ongoing relationships with travel companies can help make changes without penalty, Becky Powell, President of the Pro-Travel International,

Laurel Brunvoll, the owner of Unforgettable Voyages travel agency, recommends taking a wait and see approach to the cancellation of know how the situation plays out.

"For areas with increased risk, while this may depend on when someone is planning to travel there,"

If you go ahead with a trip

Perhaps it would be too expensive to cancel. Maybe that travelers will not just reschedule, they are not in a high-risk group, and the destination is not under aboard. Whatever the reason, the trip is still on the table.

'Experts say the key before going to prepare in case the situation changes'

"I think if you are going to travel and I do not say this is a bad idea, I would like to take a vacation myself, I think people should be aware that there is a possibility that you might get stuck somewhere for a long time, "said Watson.

CHAPTER 9: WHAT YOU NEED TO KNOW ABOUT CORONAVIRUSES

Bc coronavirus has made Italy a level 3 "do not travel if you can help" area myself. My sister and my mother called to see where we can go instead of Italy lol.

March 1, 2020

She said during a trip, and travelers should monitor new changes and adjust their behavior accordingly if the disease runs in a community staying away from public places, anyone who appears sick and large gatherings of people.

Some countries restrict where people can go or if someone is allowed into the affected areas, which could interfere with travel plans. Popular attractions may not be open; Louvre closed on Sunday and the Disney theme parks in Shanghai, Hong Kong, and Tokyo while temporarily closed.

A sign informs people about the closure of the Louvre Museum in Paris, March 2 (Adrienne SURPRISE-Nant / Bloomberg News)

Tony Rocca-forte, the chief adviser of security at the World risk management company Aware, said in an email that travelers must build redundancy into their plans, adding the time delays and preparing to improvise if conditions change.

"Make backups of your backups for all your communication devices, batteries, food/water, medication/eyeglasses, financial tools, transportation, lodging, plane tickets, etc. ", he said.

Before leaving, he said, vacationers should get all their ducks in a house behind the line: update their wills and powers of attorney, confirm the life insurance and health insurance and update their International file vaccination. Travelers should create a detailed itinerary of where they will be and when to give a colleague or a trusted person at home.

What are the chances that you get sick of being on a plane?

Erika Richter, the spokesman for the American Society of Travel Advisors, said in an email that travelers might consider putting the work equipment with them in case they end up marooned and should bring extra copies of passport, itinerary and proof of insurance.

Watson said the recommendation is that people have 30 days of prescription drugs with them, and they should also bring their original prescription in case they need more on the road.

Anyone who is sick should not travel not only to avoid spreading the disease but also to prevent being pulled out of line and potentially quarantined, said Quigley, International SOS.

He said carefully wipe the moving surfaces is "always in order," because many viruses and bacteria can survive on objects. The CDC said it might be possible for a person to get the coronavirus by touching something that has the virus and then touching your mouth, nose, or eyes, but it is not yet known how long the virus can survive on surfaces.

The bases are crucial to prevent infection, Courtney Kansler, senior health information analyst world Aware.

"This frequently includes with soap hand washing and water or use a sanitizer alcohol-based hand rub if soap and water are not available," she said. "Use social distancing and avoiding sick people.

Transit quickly in airports and transportation hubs in the same crowded. "

Travelers who had not bought travel insurance when they booked a trip should consider adding a medical policy before going out, Barto square mouth said that the coverage is limited. She said last week that nearly a third of suppliers on the site offer coverage that would include the virus.

I am genuinely concerned about the coronavirus, but I'm also worried about the insane amount of money that my mother and I will not return if travel is entirely closed in the following month.

Jacqueline February 28, 2020

If you see the future Travel

For some travelers, no virus spread will be enough to stifle Wanderlust, especially with spring break and the season of the summer holiday approaches.

So how to proceed?

There are travel advisories and official warnings about where not to go. And the maps show where the spread of the virus. But experts warn against simply choose a place that has not seen a confirmed case.

"Every day we see reports of an increasing number of countries its first cases of the virus, and in addition to this, we see the countries known to have the virus report an increase," Bogoch said, the specialist in infectious diseases research co-author in the spread of the virus."If we are not calling this pandemic, at least we are sitting on the precipice of an epidemic. "

Quigley said it is essential for travelers always to look to be applied regulations and rules wherever they go and achieve everything that could change if and when the World Health Organization declared a pandemic.

"The answers everything will be different, but there will be a significant impact on both domestic travel and across borders," he said.

Travelers considering where to go potential consequences need factors for the spread of the virus' in their decision-making, Rocca-forte said, of the world is aware. He said that includes the possibility of quarantines, travel restrictions, bans on public transport, water and food rationing, social unrest, and strained health systems.

Anyone traveling should think about what they would find medical attention if pain or sick.

"This is more important for people who have underlying health problems, and becomes even more important if an infectious disease outbreak occurs," Watson said the Johns Hopkins Center for Health Safety.

Making those plans now can still buy insurance if they decide after canceling due to fears of coronavirus, but the policy will not be cheap.

"Right now, the only and best option we recommend for people is a 'cancel for any reason' policy," Barto said. He said that which is only available within the first 10 to 21 days of booking a trip costs about 40 percent more than standard cancellation policy. It reimburses 75 percent of the cost of the trip.

Richter, the spokesman for the American Society of Travel Advisors, suggests using a professional to help make plans for spring or summer.

"A travel consultant can help you through your list of options and prices that can help you come up with a plan A, B, and C and have those options backup on hand talk can put your mind at ease.

"In times like these, a defender of travel is required."

Economic forecasts
global growth

The financial situation remains very fluid. Uncertainty about the duration and depth of the economic effects of the health crisis fuels the perception of risk and volatility in financial markets and corporate decision-making. Also, doubts about the global pandemic and effectiveness of public policies to limit its spread add to the volatility of the market.

Compounding the economic situation is a historic fall in the price of crude oil, reflecting the overall decline in economic activity prospects for disinflation. It contributes to the deterioration of the global economy through various channels. On April 29, 2020, Federal Reserve Chairman Jay Powell said the Federal Reserve could use its "full range of tools" to support economic activity as the Commerce Department reported a 4.8% drop in GDP EE .S. in the first quarter of 2020. was assessing the state of the U.S. economy, the Federal Open Market Committee issued a statement saying that "public health crisis underway in the short term and poses profoundly on economic activity, employment and inflation burden significant risks to the economic outlook in the medium term. "

The Organization for Economic Co-operation and Development (OECD), on March 2, 2020, I reduced its forecast for global economic growth at 0.5% for 2020 from 2.9% to 2.4%, based on the assumption that the economic effects of the virus would peak in the first quarter of 202016. However, the OECD estimates that if the economic impact of the disease does not arise in the first quarter, it is now clear that it was not, global economic growth would increase by 1.5% in 2020. this forecast seems now to have been very optimistic.

On March 23, 2020, the Secretary-General of the OECD, Angel Gurria, said:

The magnitude of the current shock introduces unprecedented complexity for economic forecasting. The Interim Economic Outlook OECD, published on March 2, 2020, made the first attempt to take stock of the likely impact of COVID-19 on global growth. Still, it seems that we have moved beyond even the most severe scenario than expected pandemic. It has also launched a major economic crisis that will burden our societies in the coming years.

On March 26, 2020, the OECD revised its global economic forecast based on the continuing effects of the pandemic, and governments have adopted measures to contain the spread of the virus. According to the updated estimate, measures current containment could reduce global GDP of 2.0% per month, or an annual rate of 24%, approaching the level of economic contraction not experienced since the Great Depression of the decade 1930. the OECD estimates will be revised when the OECD releases updated data specific to the country.

Labeling the expected decline in global economic activity as the "Great Lockdown," the IMF released a forecast updated on April 14, 2020. The IMF concluded that the global economy could experience its "worst recession since the Great Depression, beating observed during the Global financial crisis a decade "The IMF estimated that the worldwide economy could decline by 3.0% in 2020 before growing by 5.8% in 2021 ago, it is expected that world trade to fall in 2020 11.0% and is expected to oil prices falling by 42%.

This assumes that the prognosis pandemic fades in the second half of 2020 and that containment measures can be reversed quickly.

The IMF also noted that many countries face multiple layers, including a health crisis, an internal economic crisis, a fall in external demand, capital outflows, and a fall in raw materials prices. In combination, these various effects are interacting in ways that make the prediction difficult.

Are advanced forecast economies as a group to experience an economic contraction in 2020 of 7.8% of GDP, with the U.S. economy by the IMF projected to decline by 5.9%, almost twice the rate decline experienced in 2009 during the financial crisis, as indicated. The price of economic growth in the eurozone is expected to decline by 7.5% of GDP. It is anticipated that most developing economies and emerging experience a decrease in the rate of economic growth of 2.0%, reflecting the tightening of global financial conditions and falling prices trade and commodities throughout the world. By contrast, China, India, and Indonesia are expected to experience low but favorable economic growth rates in 2020. The IMF also argues that the recovery of the global economy could be weaker than expected due to persistent uncertainty on a possible contagion, lack of confidence, and the permanent closure of companies and changes in companies and households.

Before the COVID-19 pop, the world economy was struggling to regain a broad-based recovery as a result of the continuing impact of rising trade protectionism, trade disputes between major trading partners, falling prices of raw materials and energy, and economic uncertainty in Europe over the effect of the withdrawal of the U.K. from the European Union. Individually, each of these topics presented a solvable challenge for the world economy. Altogether, however, the problems weakened the global economy and reducing the policy flexibility of many national leaders, especially among the major developed economies available. In this environment, COVID-19.

You could have a considerable impact. While the level of economic effects over time becomes more explicit, the response to the pandemic could have a significant effect and last in the way companies organize their workforces, global supply chains, and how governments respond to a health crisis worldwide.

The OECD estimates that direct and indirect economic costs increased by global supply chains. The demand for goods and services and lower tourist and business trips decreased mean that "the negative consequences of these developments in other countries (non-OECD) are important." World trade measured by trading volume slowed in the last quarter of 2019 and is expected in 2020 related to the pandemic due to the weaker global economy are declining, in different areas harms economic activity, including airlines, hospitality, sports, and marine industry.

According to OECD forecasts updated:

The most significant impact confinement restrictions will be on retail and wholesale trade, professional services, and real estate, although there are substantial differences between countries.

closures could reduce economic output in advanced countries and major emerging economies by 15% or more; other emerging economies could experience a drop in production of 25%.

countries that depend on tourism could be affected more severely, while countries with agricultural and mining sectors could suffer less severe effects.

The economic impacts are likely to vary between countries reflect differences in the timing and degree of containment measures.

Also, the OECD says that China's emergence as a global economic player marks a significant departure from previous comprehensive health episodes. China's growth, combined with globalization and interdependence of economies through capital flows, supply chains, and foreign investment, magnifies the cost of the spread of the virus through quarantines and restricted mobility of labor and travel.

The global economic role of China and globalization mean that trade plays a role in the dissemination of economic effects Covid-19.

More generally, the economic impact of the pandemic spreads through three sales channels:

1. by supply chains that the reduced economic activity covered by producers of intermediate goods to finished goods producers.
2. due to an overall decline in economic activity, reducing demand for products in general, including imports.
3. by reduced trade with commodity exporters that supply producers, who, in turn, reduced their imports and negatively affects the trade and economic activity of the exporters.

Global trade

By April 8, 2020, provided by the World Trade Organization (WTO), it is expected that the volume of world trade will decline between 13% and 32% by 2020 as a result of the economic impact of COVID-19, WTO, as shown in Table 2, found the entire spectrum of the high level of uncertainty in forecasting the Treasury in terms of duration and economic impact of the pandemic and actual is outside this range could result, and more upper or lower.

Most optimistic scenario assumes that WTO trade volumes recover quickly in the second half of 2020 to its previous trend pandemic, or that the world economy is recovering as V. The most pessimistic scenario assumes a partial recovery which lasts until 2021 or suffering from the global economic activity over improvement in the form of U. The WTO concluded that the impact on the volume of world trade could surpass the fall of world trade during the height of the financial crisis of 2008-2009.

Estimates show that all geographic regions will experience a decline in the double-digit trading volume for "other regions," which from Africa, the Middle East, and the Commonwealth of Independent States with the exception. North America and Asia would experience the most significant declines in export volumes. The forecast also projects that sectors with high-value chains such as automotive products and electronics could suffer the most significant reductions.

Although services are not included in the forecast of the WTO, this segment of the economy could suffer the most significant changes as a result of restrictions on travel and transport and closing commercial establishments and hospitality. However, services such as information technology are growing to meet the demand of employees working from home.

Economic policy challenges

The challenge for the authorities has been implementing specific policies to deal with the expected short-term problems without creating distortions in the economy that survive the virus's effects. However, policymakers are being overtaken by the rapidly changing nature of the global health crisis that seems to be becoming a world trade and the economic crisis, whose effects on the economy worldwide are increasing.

As the economic impact of the pandemic grows, the authorities are giving more weight to policies that address the immediate financial consequences at the expense of long-term considerations, such as debt accumulation. Initially, many politicians had felt limited To respond in their ability the crisis as a result of the limited flexibility of monetary and fiscal support in conventional standards, given the synchronized slowdown broad-based global economic growth, particularly in the manufacture and trade that had developed viral outbreak.

The pandemic is also affecting global politics, and global leaders are canceling international meetings28, and some nations.

According to reports, they are fueling conspiracy theories that blame other countries.

Initially, it was expected that the economic effects of the virus to be Supply problems in the short term as a factory were issued because workers were to reduce the spread of the virus through social interaction quarantined.

The decline in economic activity, initially in China, has had international repercussions as companies experienced delays in deliveries of intermediate and finished goods through the supply chain.

Raise concerns, however, that the supply shock related virus is creating demand shocks longer and far-reaching as reduced activity by consumers and businesses have a lower rate of economic growth. As demand shocks are developed, companies are experiencing reduced activity, increased benefits, and potentially binding credit constraints and liquidity.

While manufacturing companies are experiencing crashes and supply chains, reduced consumer activity through social distancing affects the service sector of the economy, accounting for two-thirds of

the U.S. annual economic output. In this environment, manufacturing and service companies have tended to treasure money in cash, which affects market liquidity. In response, central banks have cut interest rates when possible and extended loan services to provide liquidity to financial markets and the company may be insolvent.

The longer the economic impact is made, the higher the economic impact should the results be transferred from commercial and financial relations with an ever-larger group of countries, companies, and households. Potentially increase this growing economic impact of liquidity constraints and credit market in the global financial markets attracting businesses to accumulate cash, with adverse effects on economic growth fallout. At the same time, the financial markets to an increase in bond issuance by the Government of factoringUnited States, Europe, and other places such as public debt levels increased to meet expected spending obligations during an economic downturn expected to increase.

Fiscal spending to combat the effects of the COVID-19.

Unlike the 2008-2009 financial crisis, reduced consumer demand, labor market issues, and a lower level of activity among enterprises,

instead of risky trading by banks worldwide, led to corporate credit problems and potential bankruptcy. These market dynamics have led some observers to question whether these events Scale Full-financial crisis marks the beginning of a global.

Market liquidity and credit policy questions were several different challenges to face supply shortages. As a result, the focus has government policy has expandable from a health crisis to the problems of macroeconomic and financial market through a combination of monetary, fiscal, and others, including border closures, quarantines, and restrictions on social interactions.

In essence, while businesses are trying to worker issues and address output at the company level, national leaders are trying to implement fiscal policies to prevent economic growth fell sharply for helping workers and businesses facing economic tensions, and central banks are adapting monetary policy to the problems of the credit market steering assembly.

In the initial phase of the health, crisis households experienced not the same kind of loss of wealth, which they saw during the financial crisis of 2008-2009 when the value of their primary residence drastically reduced. However, with numbers rapidly increasing unemployment, job losses could lead to mortgage defaults and delinquencies in payment of rent, unless financial institutions provide loan tolerance or a mechanism to provide financial assistance. In turn, the mortgage defaults could adversely affect the market for mortgage-backed securities, the availability of mortgage funds, and negatively affect the overall rate of economic growth. Losses in the value of most stock markets in the US, Asia, and Europe could also affect household wealth, especially retirees living on a fixed income and others who own shares.

Investors trading mortgage-backed securities reports have been reducing their holdings while the Federal Reserve has been trying to support it.31 In the current environment, including traditional policy instruments such as monetary accommodation at the seem, have not been conventionally processed by the markets, with indices of the stock market Displaying increased, rather than the lower levels, uncertainty after the Federal Reserve cut interest rates, the volatility Such is adding to doubts about what governments can do to address deficiencies in the global economy.

Economic Developments

Between late February and April 2020, the financial markets of the United States to Asia and Europe have already been whipsawed investors have grown concerned that COVID-19 would create the economic and financial crisis overall with indicators to indicate how long and extensive economic effects can be.32 investors searched for investment haven, as the benchmark U.S. Treasury security ten years, experienced a record drop in yield below 1%, March

3 2020.33 in response to concerns that the global economy was in a freefall, the Fed reduced interest rates on March 3, 2020, to support economic activity, while the Bank of Japan spent on shopping assets to provide short-term liquidity to Japanese banks; The Government of Japan indicated that it would also help workers with wage subsidies.

The Bank of Canada also cut its first interest rate. The International Monetary Fund (IMF) announced that it was about $ 50 trillion available through emergency financing facilities for low-income and emerging countries and funds available through its containment disaster and relief Trust (CCRT).

The uncertainty of investors, the Dow Jones Industrial Average (DJIA) lost equivalent to about a third of its value between February 14, 2020, and March 23, 2020, the expectation that the U.S. Congress could be a package of $ 2.0 trillion spending Dow Jones will have shifted by more than 11% on March 24, 2020 move from March 23 to April 15 Dow Jones higher by18%. Since then, the Dow Jones has moved erratically as investors weighed news about the human cost and economic impact of the pandemic and prospects of various medical treatments. For some politicians, the fall in stock prices has raised concerns that foreign investors could try to take advantage of the situation by increasing the purchases of companies in sectors that are considered national security as necessary. Ursula von der Leyen, President of the European Commission, called for E.U.. members to better screen foreign investment, especially in areas such as health, medical research, and infrastructure.35 similar criticism to the global financial crisis of 2008-2009, the central banks have implemented several monetary transactions to provide liquidity to their economies.

These actions, however, were initially not entirely positive by all participants in the financial market that questioned the use of policy instruments of central banks, which are similar to those employed during the financial crisis of 2008-2009, despite the current crisis this is fundamentally different in origin.

In the last financial crisis, central banks intervened to restart lending and spending of banks that had participated in risky assets. In the current environment, central banks are trying to cope with the volatility of the financial market and prevent large-scale reflect underlying economic uncertainty caused by the pandemic business insolvencies.

A the same as in the conditions during the financial crisis of 2008-2009, the dollar has become the preferred currency by investors, reinforcing its role as a dominant reserve currency world, the dollar rose more than 3.0% during the period March 3y 13,

2020, reflecting the increase in international demand for the dollar and dollar-denominated assets. From their highs on March 23, the dollar has given up some of its value against other currencies but has remained around 10% higher than it was at the beginning of the year.

A recent survey conducted by the Bank for International Settlements (BIS) represents $ 36 for 88% of the global turnover of the foreign exchange market. It is crucial in financing a series of financial transactions, including serving as an invoicing currency to facilitate international trade. It also represents two-thirds of foreign exchange reserves of central banks, half of the foreign currency deposits of the non-US bank, and two-thirds of non-US corporate loans from banks and corporate bond markets.37 As a result, interruptions in the functioning of the world market for the dollar may have a far-reaching impact on international trade and financial proceedings.

The international role of the dollar also increases the pressure on the Federal Reserve to necessarily assume the lead role as a global lender of last resort. Reminiscent of the financial crisis, the world economy has experienced a period of shortage of dollars, requiring the Federal Reserve to take numerous measures to ensure the supply of dollars to the U.S. and global economies, including activation of existing currency swap contracts, the establishment of such new agreements with central banks, and the creation of new financial services to provide liquidity to central banks

monetary authorities.38 Generally, banks lend long-term and short-term loan and can only borrow from their local central bank. In turn, central banks can only provide liquidity in the currency.

Consequently, a bank can not cash in a panic, which means that it can borrow in private markets to meet cash flow needs in the short term. Swap lines are designed to allow foreign central banks to provide the necessary liquidity to banks in their country in dollars.

The bond yields of the U.S. Treasury fell to historic lows on March 6, 2020. March 9, 2020, as investors continue to move out of stocks and securities of the Treasury and other government securities, including the U.K. and German bonds were due to concerns about the impact of the pandemic in part on the growth and economic expectations that the Federal Reserve and other central banks short-term interest rates.39 could cut on March 5, U.S. Congress approved an expenditure of $ 8Billion bills to health aid, sick, small business loans and international cooperation. At the same time, prices of raw materials declined sharply as a result of reduced economic activity and disagreements among producers of more cuts oil production of crude oil and lower global demand for commodities, including oil raw.

CONCLUSION

This book explains about the world situation and the impact based on the global economy on Covid-19, teach us the skills on how to use a face mask and describe and list how to make a face mask in different type with a simple step to protect and give information about social boost, the impact it has had on tourism and the situation in travel and holidays.

www.ingramcontent.com/pod-product-compliance
Lightning Source LLC
Chambersburg PA
CBHW070756250726
48662CB00004B/1835